ALLEN PHOTOGRAPHIC GUIDES

YOUR
HORSE'S FEET

CONTENTS

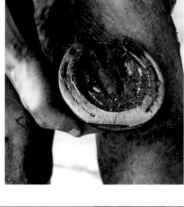

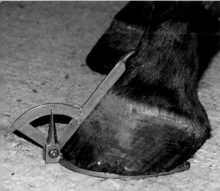

THE HORSE'S FOOT

STRUCTURE AND FUNCTION

The horse's foot has evolved over fifty million years from the four toes of Hyracotherium (*Eohippus*), a tiny browsing animal (*see right*), to the single hoof of *Equus*, a much larger plains-dwelling animal. The evolutionary changes are thought to be related to the need to run fast in order to escape from predators and the mechanics of an increase in the size of the animal. The splint bones of the modern horse are the vestigial remains of the extra toes.

In looking at the structure of the horse's foot we cannot ignore the rest of the limb, as the conformation of the one has a great effect on the other. The bones of the fore and hind limbs are shown in the photographs below and

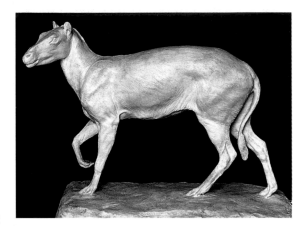

opposite (*top*). It can be seen that there are two bones in the horse's foot – the pedal (or coffin) bone and the tiny navicular bone. The joint between the short pastern and these two bones is also within the foot. This is often referred to as the 'coffin joint' and can be a source of lameness. The deep digital flexor tendon is attached to the pedal bone and can rotate it out of position if the laminae at the front of the foot are damaged. There is a large rubbery structure under these structures and above the frog called the digital cushion. This forms a shock absorber for the horse's foot and limb.

The external features of the weight-bearing surface of the hoof are shown in the photo and diagram opposite (*bottom*). The weight should be borne mainly on the hoof wall (outside the white line) and the bars and frog. The sole should be concave and take very little weight. If it becomes dropped or has a build-up of false sole or debris it can become bruised. This can also happen on very stony or rough, frozen ground. The white line is the visible junction between the hoof wall and the sensitive tissue above the sole.

The microstructure of the horse's foot is a modified version of skin. The horn of the hoof wall is an organised network of tiny tubules which give it its strength. Disruption of this structure occurs in hoof disease.

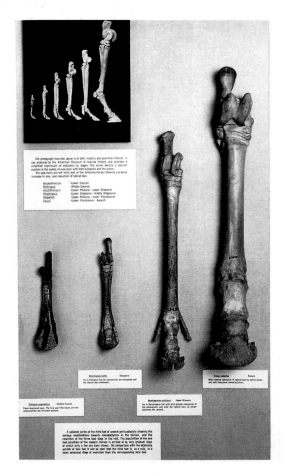

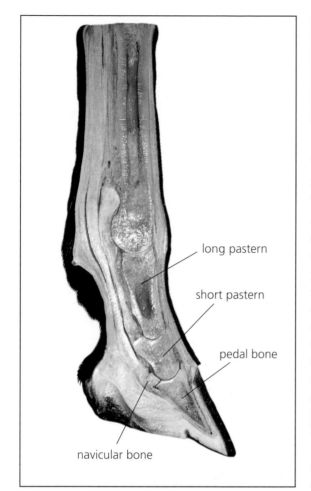

long pastern

short pastern

pedal bone

navicular bone

GROWTH

The hoof grows from the coronary band downwards taking between nine and twelve months to reach the toe and a little less to the heel.

CONFORMATION AND FOOT BALANCE

The conformation of the limb and the balance of the foot make a vital contribution to the soundness of the horse. Good farriery from an early age can do much to assist this. Severe problems may need surgery but many faults may be gradually corrected by careful trimming or remedial shoeing. Attempting to over-correct however can cause repercussions in another part of the limb. Front and hind feet differ in shape – hind ones are more elongated and have steeper walls at the inner and outer quarters. It is normal for them to turn out very slightly and the sole is slightly more concave, but each pair should be symmetrical.

Look at the horse from either side with it standing square (the leg being examined should be vertical). An imaginary line from

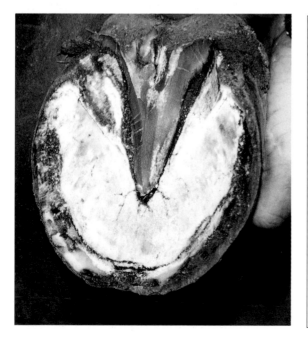

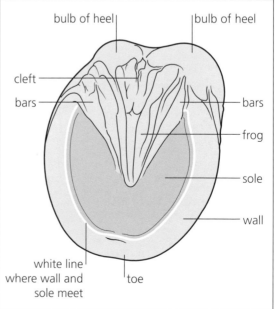

bulb of heel

bulb of heel

cleft

bars

bars

frog

sole

wall

white line where wall and sole meet

toe

the centre of the fetlock joint through the middle of the pastern ideally should be parallel to the front wall of the hoof. This line should form an angle of approximately 50° to 55° with the ground at the toe. It is believed that very upright feet may predispose to jarring and joint injuries whereas very sloping feet and pasterns may put more strain on the back tendons, particularly if the toe is allowed to get too long. If the hoof–pastern axis is not straight it may be described as broken forward (where the hoof is steeper than the pastern: *see below*) or broken back (where the pastern is more upright than the hoof: see *below right*). This may be the natural conformation of the

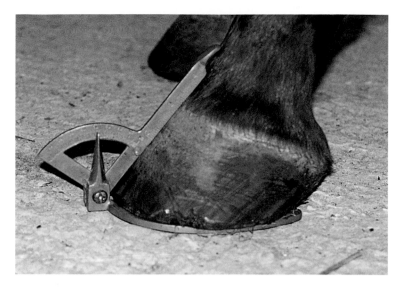

horse or due to excess horn at the toe or heel respectively. Corrective trimming will help in these cases.

Look at the horse from the front. An imaginary line through the forearm, knee, cannon

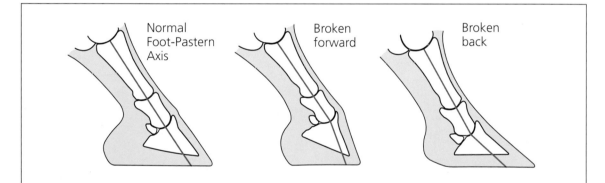

Normal Foot-Pastern Axis

Broken forward

Broken back

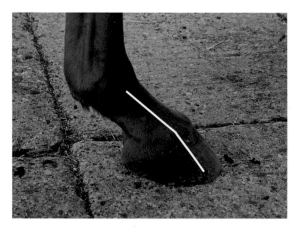

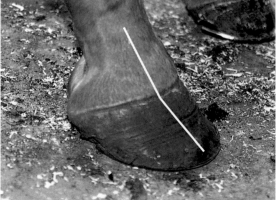

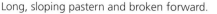

Long, sloping pastern and broken forward.

Broken back.

bone and toe should be vertical with appropriate separation of the hooves. The horse may be 'base wide', 'base narrow', 'base normal', 'pigeon toed' or 'toed out'. Symmetry is again important. Look at the horse directly from behind. *Make sure you are out of kicking range!*

Again the limbs should be vertical, although slight cow-hocks (when the hocks turn in towards each other) are acceptable in young horses. Other problems can arise from flat feet, boxy feet, club feet, contracted heels, sheared heels and dropped soles.

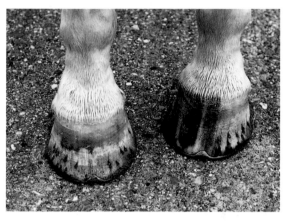

'Pigeon toed'.

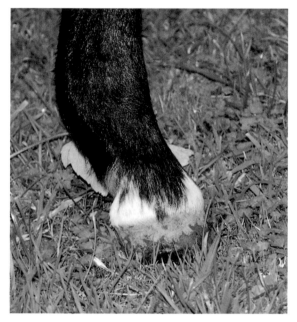

Club foot.

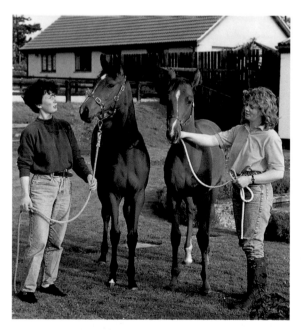

The horse on the left is 'base narrow', and the one on the right 'base normal'.

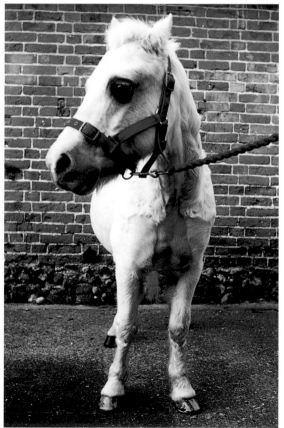

'Base wide' and 'toed out'.

The bearing surface of the hoof should be flat and symmetrical. Excess horn at one side or the other can cause wry feet (*below*) and sometimes sheared heels (*right*). If the limb is held by the pastern and the hoof allowed to hang down naturally, the bearing surface can be viewed from directly above to check that all is well (*bottom*).

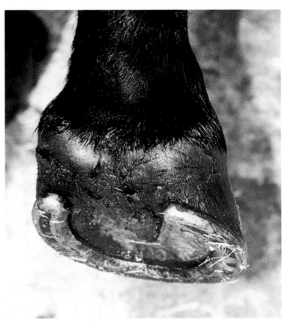

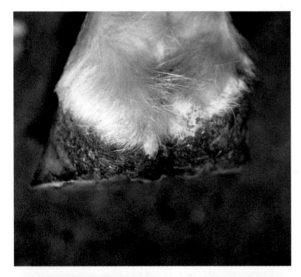

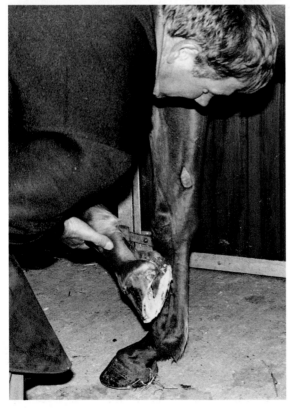

MAINTENANCE OF A HEALTHY FOOT

The horse's hoof is continually growing from the coronet and being worn away at the bearing surface. In the wild these two effects generally balance out. Unshod horses in domestic situations may be on softer ground and the hooves will become excessively long, flared, cracked or broken (*see the examples on page 7*). If ridden unshod on roads they may become overworn and make the animal footsore. The speed and quality of hoof growth is partially genetic but is also closely correlated with nutrition. Small rings or ridges in the hoof wall, parallel to the coronet, indicate changes in speed of growth. There is often a particularly clear ring which appears corresponding to the time of turnout or to a flush of spring grass (*see page 7, bottom left*). If the rings diverge at the heel this is often a sign of chronic laminitis and faster growth of horn at the heel (*see page 7, bottom right*).

A normal balanced diet should be adequate for healthy feet but because of the delayed effect people sometimes forget to provide this all the year round. A good example of this is during the late autumn when the grass may not

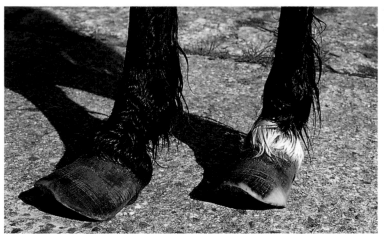

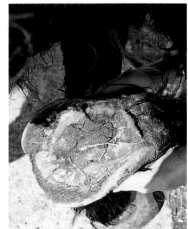

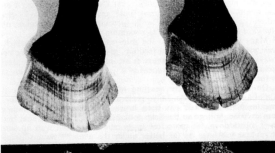

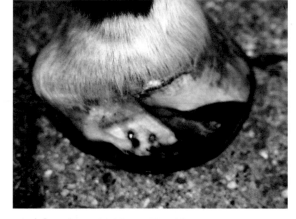

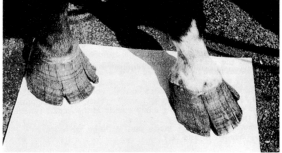

Top left and top right Long, flared hooves.
Left Badly cracked hooves. *Above* A broken hoof.

Below left A clearly visible ring. *Below right* Rings
divergent at heel, a sign of laminitis.

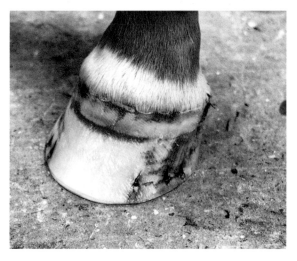

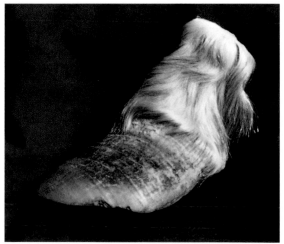

be very nutritious. About nine months later, in mid or late summer, the horse's feet become brittle and crumbly, and shoes are lost. The hoof formed when nutrition was poor has now reached the bearing surface and nail-holding areas. Dry conditions and hard ground may aggravate the situation.

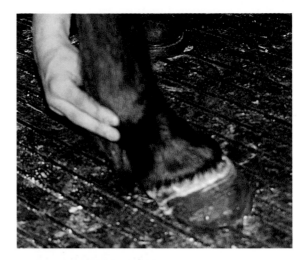

COMMON PROBLEMS AND DISEASES

Detecting hoof pain can involve feeling for heat, checking for an increased digital pulse, observing the horse's gait when walking, trotting and turning.

WARNING

If animals are severely lame then move them as little as possible.

If it is suspected that the source of pain is in the foot, then hoof testers may be used to find whether one area of the foot is more sensitive than others. This may give further clues as to where to look more closely for pus or bruising. Some horses are more sensitive than others to the hoof testers. If necessary make comparisons with the sound foot. If an area of pain is confirmed then examine it closely. You may need to remove the shoe at this stage. This is something that all able-bodied, competent owners can learn to do and only requires basic tools. (*See pages 18, 19.*)

Pus

Pus in the foot is one of the commonest causes of lameness in the horse and one of the

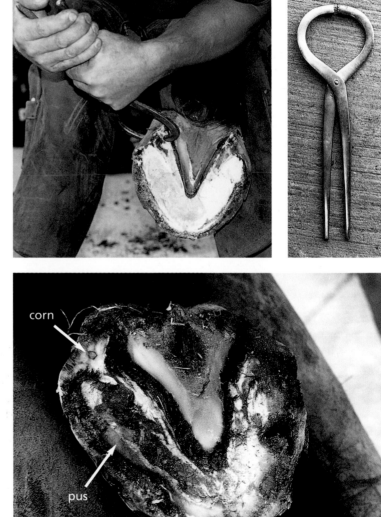

corn

pus

most easily relieved. It is usually caused by a foreign body, often gravel or occasionally a nail, getting into (*prick*) or close to (*nail bind*) the sensitive part of the hoof and being sealed off. An abscess forms and the horse becomes lame, sometimes so severely that the leg is almost non-weight-bearing. As the hoof is unable to swell it is very painful for the horse (imagine having a thorn under your finger nail). Competent owners can undertake a preliminary investigation. Carefully examine the sole of the foot using a sharp hoof pick or preferably a hoof knife to scrape the surface. Any small black marks or signs of a penetrating wound should be carefully investigated to see if they track into the hoof. Very often if they can be opened up, black pus will ooze out and the horse will be much improved within hours. Many vets prefer not to give antibiotics as this can lead to a grumbling abscess which recurs later. Occasionally the pus will work its way upwards and appear at the coronet. This may be the first sign of infection, or it may be because there has been inadequate downwards drainage. Such cases should always be seen by a vet to prevent complications.

Poulticing

Where pus in the foot is suspected or has been found, poulticing is often recommended to ensure removal of all infected matter or to soften the foot to enable release of pus. The traditional method of poulticing was to use wet bran and sacking to form a boot over the hoof. There are a variety of poultice boots on the market. Kaolin or Epsom salts (magnesium sulphate) could also be used. It is much better to use a commercially available poultice such as Animalintex, which is effective and clean and enables any exudate to be examined. The poultice should be soaked according to the manufacturer's instructions and placed over the suspect area. This should then be covered with padding and polythene to prevent it from drying out. (The photos show the materials for and the application of a poultice.) The

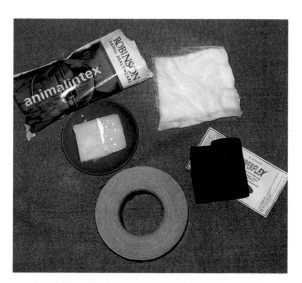

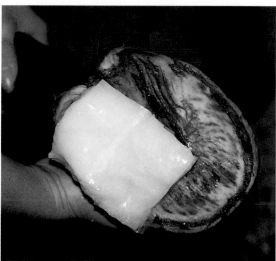

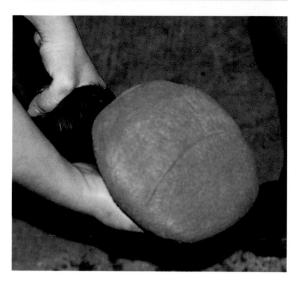

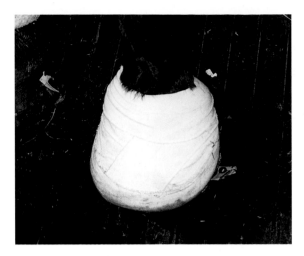

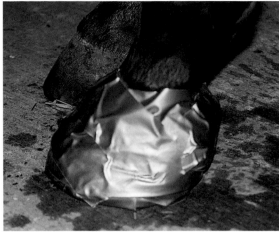

poultice may be held on with bandaging or tape. A cheap way is to use grey elephant or duct tape, which moulds easily into a protective cover and is available in big rolls from DIY stores. The poultice should be changed twice a day to begin with, but later may be left for 24 hours. Tubbing the foot twice a day with warm water and Epsom salts may also help. If there is not rapid relief then consult your veterinary surgeon.

CAUTION!

Although pus in the foot is very common, a fractured pedal bone which must receive veterinary treatment can cause the same symptoms.

Bruising

Bruising of the sole may show as a purplish pink area when the sole is scraped or trimmed or as corns which may be yellowish and pink. Both of these symptoms are the result of pressure or concussion. It may be mild, for example where a horse has been walking over rough, frozen or stony ground, and cause no lameness, or it may be severe enough to cause an abscess (*see page 8*). In the case of corns (*see photo on page 8*) – usually in the 'seat of corn' – they can become very deep seated and cause prolonged or intermittent lameness.

Ask your farrier for advice as he will dig them out and may recommend seating out the shoe at the heel (*see the photos below*). Be careful to keep the area free from dirt.

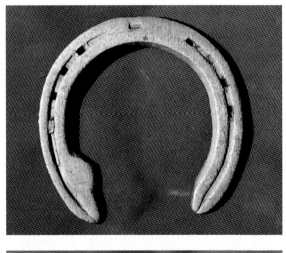

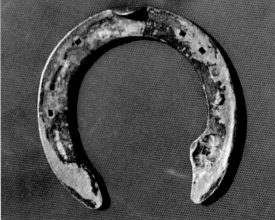

Cracks

Cracks can appear in the wall of the hoof either from stress or trauma. Small ones may be superficial and of no consequence (*see below*) but sandcracks, which start at the coronet, can make the horse lame and become worse the more the horse is used. Sometimes shoeing an unshod horse may be sufficient to control the situation. Some farriers may rasp a line across the top of the crack to prevent it from spreading, or apply a kind of staple to hold the crack together. Very severe cases may need the whole crack cut out to allow new hoof to regrow from the coronet. Fillers may be used to protect exposed areas (*see the three photos on the right*). Sometimes damage to the wall can be caused by a tread from a hoof with a stud in the shoe, or by a wire injury. These cases need veterinary advice in consultation with your farrier.

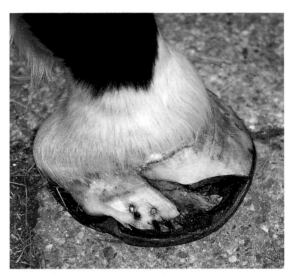

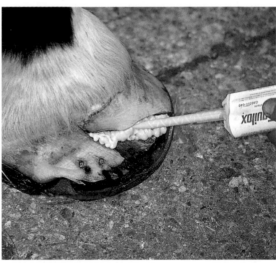

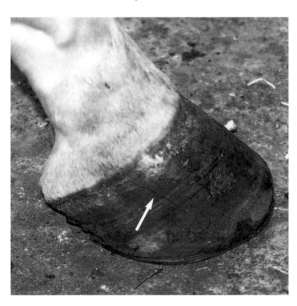

Small crack in hoof wall.

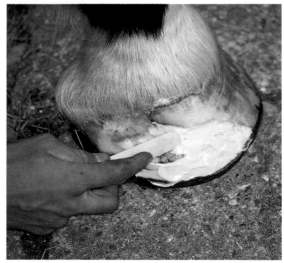

TUMOURS

Tumours of the foot are rare but keratomas are occasionally seen. They may show on the bearing surface of the foot as a displacement of the white line.

Overgrowth

Feet can become severely overgrown if neglected, particularly if the animal is only walking on soft ground, and the mobility and comfort of the horse is severely compromised. Sometimes the overgrowth is exacerbated by disease such as Cushing's Disease, not uncommon in elderly horses, where there may be an effect from a pituitary tumour. Very long curled up feet are sometimes referred to as 'Turkish slippers' (*right*). Regular trimming by a farrier, at least every eight weeks, will cause a spectacular improvement in mobility.

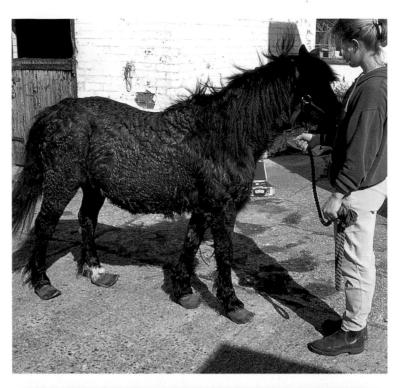

Laminitis

Laminitis is the scourge of the domestic horse world and there is an Allen Photographic Guide by Karen Coumbe dedicated to it. The commonest cause is too much spring grass, particularly in little fat ponies, but other causes include grain overload, trauma, concussion, stress from excessive weight-bearing (such as when another foot is very lame), toxaemia, retained afterbirth and administration of steroids.

There has been much discussion and research in recent years into the exact mechanism of the disease but it is now believed that substances released from the hindgut in certain conditions cause the laminae to pull apart. This is very painful for the horse and in severe cases these tissues die and tear as the pedal bone is pulled away from the inside of the wall

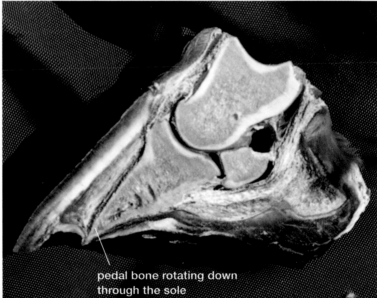

pedal bone rotating down through the sole

of the hoof by the deep digital flexor tendon (*see above*). Once this happens there is permanent damage which causes chronic lameness problems and sometimes necessitates euthanasia. Early detection and treatment is vital if the animal is to return to work.

SHOEING

Why shoe your horse? It is an expensive business and usually needs to be done every four to six weeks. If your horse is mainly working on soft surfaces such as an indoor or outdoor school or on grass, it may not need shoes, only a trim about every eight weeks. Most horses however have to do a fair amount of roadwork or work on hard ground. This means that the hoof wears down faster than it grows and the horse would become footsore or pick up gravel. The need to reshoe is governed by the hoof growth, which needs trimming back, and the wear on the shoes which will depend on the amount of roadwork done. Some horses wear their shoes unevenly owing to gait or conformation faults and they may need to be shod more frequently.

The other reasons for shoeing are to give extra grip in certain conditions or to allow studs to be used. Remedial shoes may be used to correct faults or alleviate problems such as corns, laminitis or navicular syndrome.

Basic shoes have changed little for several hundred years and are but variations on a theme of a curve of iron nailed onto the base of the hoof wall. In recent years different alloys (*below*) have been tried and glue-on shoes developed (*below right*). The first glue-on shoes

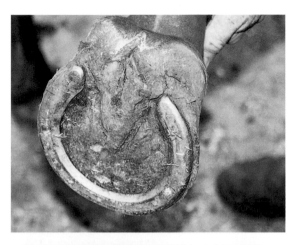

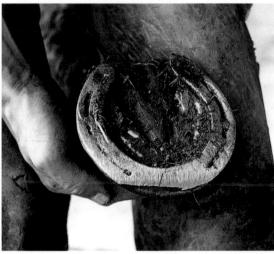

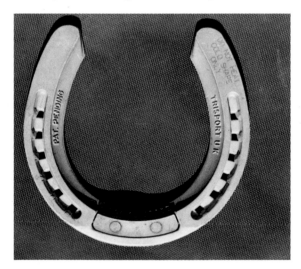

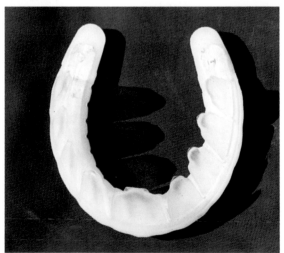

were disastrous and quickly fell off, but now excellent ones are available, if somewhat expensive. They are particularly useful where the hoof is damaged or for remedial shoes in very young animals. There are also rubber boots (*right*) which can be used as a temporary measure – for example, a lost shoe on a long-distance ride – but they are hard to keep on and they need careful fitting to prevent sore heels. These are not a new idea. In the past horses pulling lawn mowers wore thick-soled leather boots (*below*) to prevent them from damaging the turf .

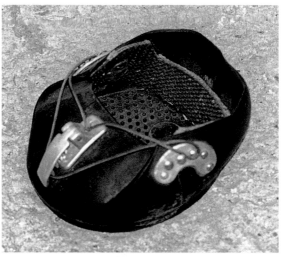

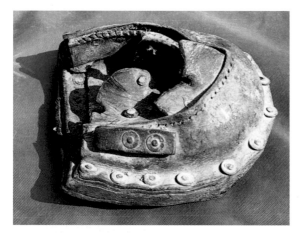

Nowadays, the commonest shoe for riding and sport horses is the 'hunter shoe' (*see below*). This is fullered for grip, concave to reduce suction, with, on the front shoes, toe clips, to prevent the foot sliding off the front, and pencilled heels, and, on the hind shoes, quarter clips and often a rolled toe to reduce the chance of damage if the horse overreaches. Traditionally there are four nail holes on the outside and three on the inside but the farrier may not use all of these.

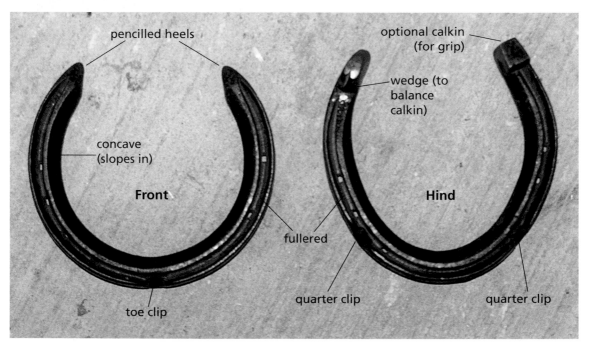

pencilled heels

optional calkin (for grip)

wedge (to balance calkin)

concave (slopes in)

Front

Hind

fullered

toe clip

quarter clip

quarter clip

SPECIAL PURPOSE, CORRECTIVE AND SURGICAL SHOEING

Many equestrian disciplines favour specialist shoes. For example, racehorses wear light-weight aluminium 'racing plates' (*right*), which tend to have more holes in them than standard shoes, as they may need putting on and taking off more frequently (between races). This gives the farrier plenty of options if the hoof wall has become damaged in places. He will use the minimum number of nails to keep the shoe on effectively.

Heavy horses traditionally wear plain stamp-ed shoes (*below*), often with calkins for grip when pulling heavy loads. They may be bev-elled to make the feet look larger for showing.

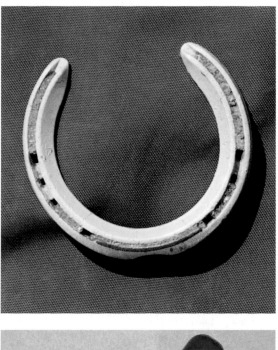

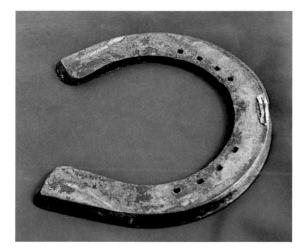

Different disciplines may have rules on studs. Racing plates, for example, are not permitted any studs or raised nail heads which could damage other horses. Polo ponies are only allowed a polo stud with no hard core and it may only be worn on the outside heel of the hind shoe within an inch of the heel.

REMEDIAL SHOES

Farriers may often be asked to produce remedial shoes for horses with a particular problem. In many cases it is just to improve foot balance, the shape of the hoof, or to change the breakover point – the point where

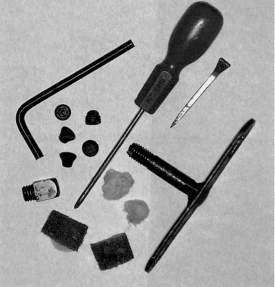

Stud fitting equipment.

the upward flight of the foot changes to forwards and downwards. They are also used to correct faulty action such as winging out (dishing), winging in and plaiting. It is impor-tant not to make very dramatic changes which might interfere with the natural way of going of the horse, as such changes could cause repercussions in other parts of the leg.

Ponies with laminitis may require frog sup-port to reduce the rotation of the pedal bone. In an emergency a roll of bandage can be strapped under the hoof but purpose made 'lily pads' (to support the frog!) are available and later the pony may be shod with a heart bar shoe. Bar shoes such as egg bars are commonly used where the frog or heels have become con-tracted, or for navicular syndrome where there is pain in the area of the navicular bone. This syndrome has been much investigated over the past few years and poor conformation and poor shoeing or foot balance are believed to be major contributory factors. Shoes are also often adapted for particular problems or injuries, for

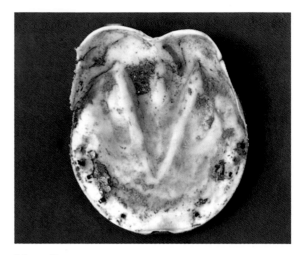

'Lily pad'.

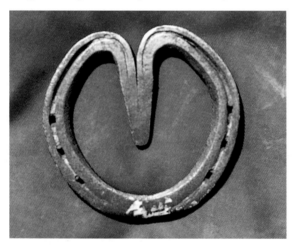

Heart bar shoe.

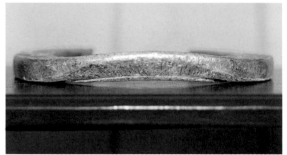

example rolled-up toes (*above*) on front shoes for horses which stumble, or toe extensions for contracted tendons to prevent knuckling over and encouraging the tendon to stretch. Lateral extensions (*below*) can improve the way a horse puts its foot down and result in

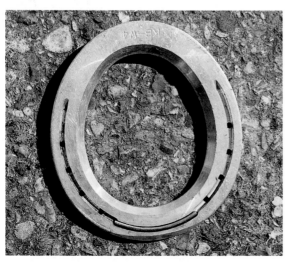

Egg bar shoe.

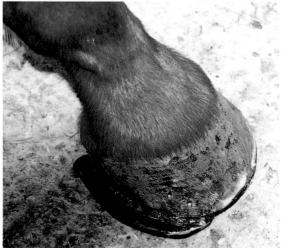

the restoration of more normal foot balance. Hospital plates are used to protect the whole of the sole of the foot where there has been a puncture injury right down to the pedal bone or something requiring surgery. Surgery involving entry into the hoof capsule must be done by a veterinary surgeon but commonly he will be working together with a specialist farrier.

In recent years the natural balance, or Fitzwygram, shoe (*below*) has become popular which enables the toe to be kept short and the heel long. This is believed to mimic the shape of the foot in wild horses, reducing stumbling and strain on tendons and ligaments, and is sometimes referred to as 'four point shoeing'.

Below and bottom left and right How hospital plates protect the foot.

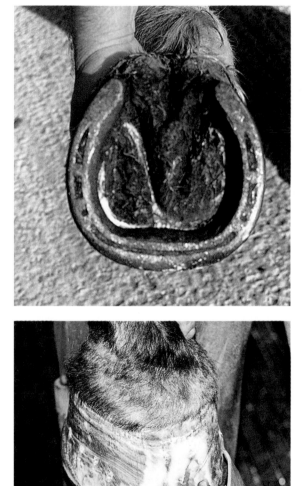

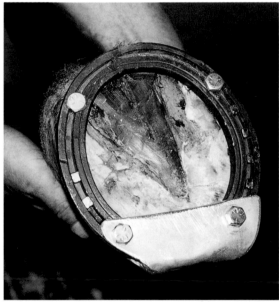

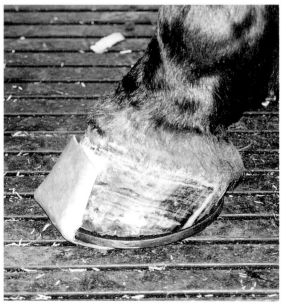

THE FARRIER

THE FARRIERS' REGISTRATION ACT 1975 (and Amendment 1977)

The Act defines farriery as the shoeing of horses including the preparation of a foot to receive a shoe. The only people in the United Kingdom who are permitted to do this are registered farriers, veterinary surgeons, and trainee farriers and veterinary students under qualified supervision. The only exception is a person rendering first aid in an emergency. (There are a few relaxations of the rules in the Highlands and Islands of Scotland where farriers are few and far between. These rules are currently under review.) A *blacksmith* is someone who works with iron but is not necessarily a registered farrier and may only do agricultural, industrial and decorative work. Farriers in the United Kingdom are registered with the Farriers' Registration Council which also has a duty to take suitable steps to prevent practice by unqualified persons. Their traditional governing body is the Worshipful Company of Farriers, an ancient Livery Company of the City of London dating back to 1356. The WCF organises and conducts examinations, prepares the syllabus, holds competitions and looks after injured or needy farriers.

There is a code of conduct between farriers and veterinary surgeons to ensure good relations. Farriers are not exempt from the Veterinary Surgeons' Act and may not diagnose, prescribe drugs or perform surgery. Most farriers and veterinary surgeons respect each other's skills and are keen to liaise with each other and work together.

TRAINING

It normally takes four years to train as a farrier. This involves being apprenticed to a recognised training farrier and spending some time on block release (27 weeks at a college spread over the four years) and taking examinations.

The basic qualification is the Diploma of the Worshipful Company of Farriers (earlier known as Registered Shoeing Smith – RSS) or the Army Trade Test BII in Farriery. Some farriers may have a higher qualification – the AWCF (Associate) or the highest – FWCF (Fellow). There are still a few farriers on a special section of the Register who have 'grandfather rights' from before the introduction of the Farriers' Registration Acts. They had not taken exams but had a number of years of practical experience.

TOOLS

Most farriers now have mobile gas-fired forges in the back of a van and are able to travel to their clients' premises to hot shoe. There are however still many traditional forges, some of which are coal-fired. Most farriers like to have access to a specialist forge where they can make hand-made and specialist shoes; this is a prerequisite for an Approved Training Farrier. Factory-made shoes, including common remedial shoes, are now available in a huge range of sizes and these can be adjusted after heating to fit most animals. It is also possible to cold shoe where only minor adjustments are needed.

First the old shoe is removed using a buffer and hammer to raise the clenches and pincers to prise off the shoe. The foot is then dressed using a combination of a drawing knife, hoof cutters and a rasp. Some farriers prefer a toeing knife which enables larger quantities of hoof to be removed at once and which, some say, produces a flatter surface. As he proceeds, the farrier will frequently check the foot balance, sometimes using a T-square. The foot may be measured at its widest point and diagonally from the quarter to the heel to estimate the size of shoe required and the farrier will select the nearest size to this. The shoe will then be heated in the forge so that adjustments may be

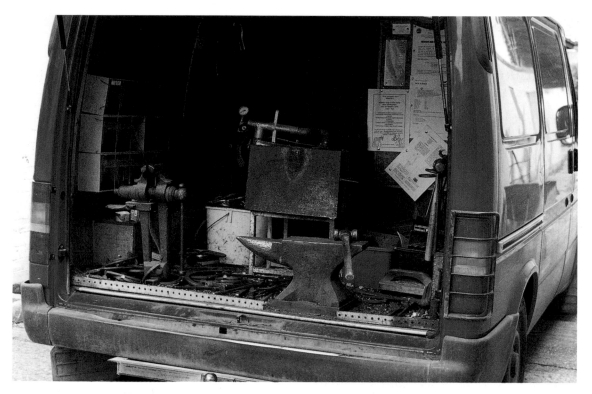

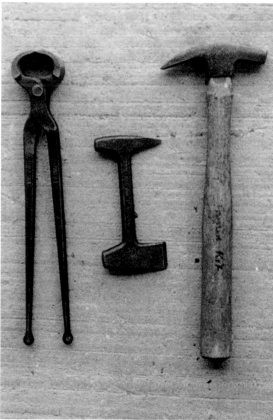

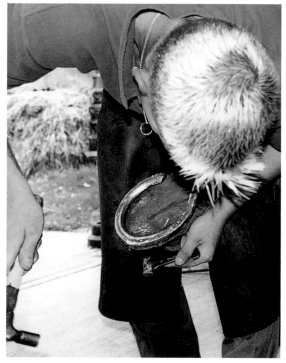

Top Nowadays most farriers have a mobile forge.

Above Raising the clenches with buffer and hammer.

Left Pincers, buffer and hammer.

made. The hot shoe is handled with tongs and a pritchel or 'hot tongs' so that it may be burnt onto the horse's foot. This produces a cloud of smoke and a hissing sound but causes the horse no pain. It enables the farrier to see how good a fit the shoe is and bed the shoe slightly into the foot ensuring a flat surface.

Once the farrier is satisfied with the fit he will plunge the shoes into cold water to cool them before nailing on. The nail heads should be chosen so that they do not stand too proud of the shoe and mainly sit in the fullering. The ends of the nails should appear in a regular line about one third of the way up the hoof wall. These ends are twisted off with the claw hammer to form a clench and the short end is pressed down with either a clenching tool or a hammer. The rough ends are smoothed off with a rasp and minor adjustments of the hoof and shoe edges may be made to give a smooth and tidy finish with no sharp edges.

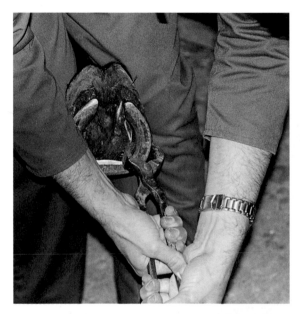

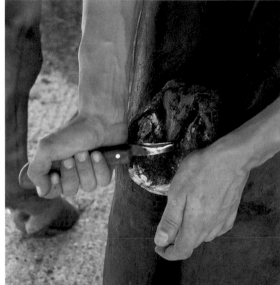

Above The old shoe is removed with pincers.

Above right The foot being dressed using a drawing knife.

Right Some farriers prefer a toeing knife.

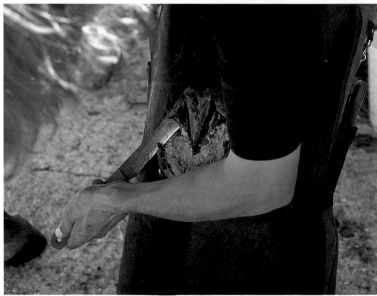

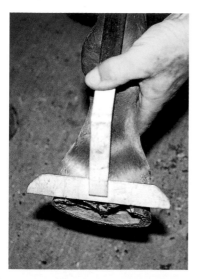

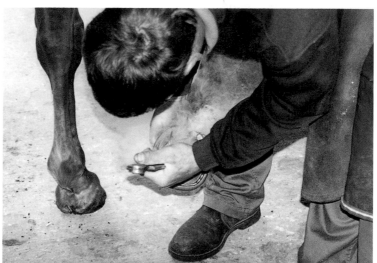

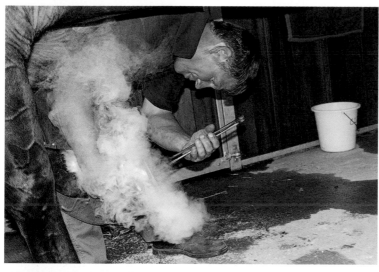

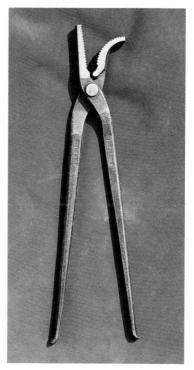

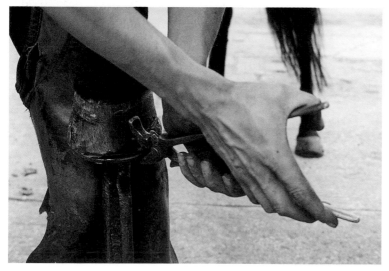

Top left Using a T-square to check the foot balance.

Top right and centre left Using 'hot tongs': the shoe is burnt onto the foot and bedded slightly into the foot to ensure a flat surface. The horse feels no pain.

Above Clenching tool.

Left Using the clenching tool.

THE HORSE OWNER'S RESPONSIBILITIES

FEEDING FOR HEALTH

Feeding a small amount of balanced concentrate daily through late autumn and winter will help to keep the feet healthy. There are also a number of feed supplements available. These need to contain a fairly high protein level as well as calcium, biotin and zinc. Read the label and check value for money. Many of these supplements and balancers are so highly advertised that more than half the price you pay goes on marketing! Alfalfa (lucerne) contains most of the requirements for healthy feet and is widely available in dried form.

The owner or rider can do much to help with the maintenance of healthy feet. Hooves should be picked out daily, particularly before and after a ride. Make sure that no stones have become lodged in the frog clefts or around the heel. If the horse is unshod check that no grit or small flints have become pressed into the sole, particularly around the white line. Any areas of flakey sole which come away easily should be scraped off to prevent the build-up of false sole which could cause pressure points. Watch out for crumbly areas (seedy toe) (*see right, above*), or black oozing liquid and a foul smell (thrush).

There are a large number of hoof dressings on the market. Some of these, for example mineral-based hoof oils, improve the appearance of the feet but should not be used too frequently as they can seal the horn off from the atmosphere. However, there are some vegetable-oil based conditioners which may benefit the condition of the hoof horn. The feet should be kept neither too wet nor too dry. During very dry periods it is helpful to wet the horse's feet daily. If there are cracks or holes, take advice from your farrier or veterinary surgeon. Hoof putties and fillers are available which are suitable for both cosmetic use and protection.

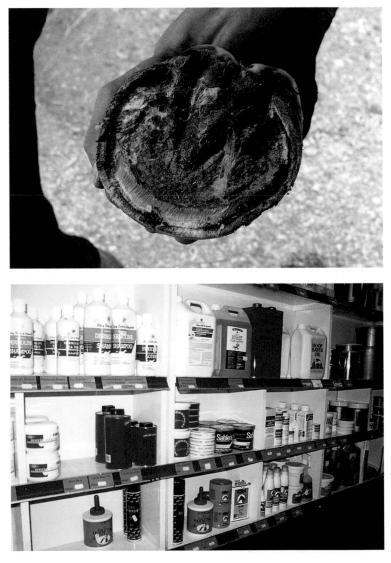

LOOKING AFTER YOUR FARRIER

It is important to maintain a good relationship with your farrier. He is bound by his trade's standards but you must play your part. Most horses need reshoeing every four to six weeks. It depends on how much work the animal is doing and on what sort of going, as well as its action. With a great deal of roadwork, shoes may be worn out in as little as two weeks. Watch for risen clenches (*right*) and loose shoes. Even if the shoes are not worn out, the foot will grow and need trimming back in about six weeks. Give the farrier plenty of notice and try to have a regular appointment with him. Make sure the horse is clean and dry, on a clean dry surface and with feet picked out. Do not expect your farrier to catch and bring your horse out of a muddy field with no one else there. Make him a cup of coffee and pay him on time! Remember, stud holes, frost nails or special shoes will cost extra. If you look after your farrier he will oblige you by coming out at short notice to replace a lost shoe, or if you have a problem. If you do not have good facilities it may be better to transport your horse to the forge or a yard where he shoes other horses. Some farriers are not keen to come to single horses so it may be easier and more flexible to join up with others in your yard. It is worth asking your vet and other horse owners in your area to help find a farrier to suit your needs.

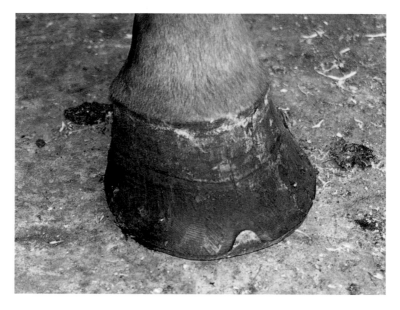

GOOD RELATIONS

In all cases it is important that there is a good and open relationship between the farrier, the owner and the veterinary surgeon.

REGISTERED FARRIERS

A list of registered farriers, together with their qualifications, can be obtained from:
The Farriers' Registration Council, Sefton House, Adams Court, Newark Road, Peterborough, Cambs, PE1 5PP.

The Worshipful Company of Farriers states that the 'well shod horse' has:

- Shoes of correct weight and size, shaped to fit the foot;

- Level feet, correct limb alignment for free movement;

- No loss of foot bearing surface;

- Clenches in a regular line, smooth and firm into the hoof wall;

- An owner who realises that foot care is his or her day-to-day responsibility too.

ACKNOWLEDGEMENTS

I am indebted to my colleagues and students at the Cambridge University
Veterinary School, the late Col. J. Hickman, farriers Martin Beadle and Chris Joyce,
Susan Beer, and as always, Mouldy.

British Library Cataloguing-in-Publication Data.
A catalogue record for this book is available from the British Library

ISBN 0.85131.828.2

© J. A. Allen 2002

Published in Great Britain in 2002 by
J. A. Allen an imprint of Robert Hale Ltd.,
Clerkenwell House, 45–47 Clerkenwell Green,
London EC1R OHT

Design and Typesetting by Paul Saunders
Edited by Susan Beer
Series editor Jane Lake
Colour processing by Tenon & Polert Colour Scanning Ltd., Hong Kong
Printed in Malta by Gutenberg Press Limited